White Cloud

Journey—

The connection of science and

medicine with philosophy and music

VOLUME II:

ACTIVATION

by

Jeffrey Fisher

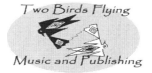

Two Birds Flying Music and Publishing

"This polarity, down through the centuries, has been observed by wisemen in esoteric traditions of both East and West. Because of it, we have consciousness, the double-edged sword with which we create or destroy. Tai chi attempts to bring about a more effective dialectic, promoting creativity as well as peace in the soul. The tai chi symbol represents this idea.

Consciousness sets us free, but it also cuts us off from that state of unquestioning participation in nature which is full of meaning. And so, we find ourselves situated at the threshold of a great void, which is our new home. The way of transforming this void into a place where human life can remain whole and integrated is called, in the Chinese tradition, the Tao. Tai Chi, at its highest order, apprehends the Tao."

--Dr. Marshall Ho'o <u>Tai Chi Chuan</u>

"Am I my brother's beeper?"

—Jeffrey Fisher, "Fractured Quotes"

WHITE CLOUD JOURNEY

OVERVIEW

VOLUME ONE:

THE TAO OF JUST ABOUT EVERYTHING

The Tao of Just About Everything is about the connection between the I-Ching, the ancient Chinese book of philosophy and divination, the genetic code and the way music is put together. We can match up not only the mathematical form and the geometric design, but also the emotional tone of musical scales with the meaning of the chapter of the I-Ching and the function of the amino acid formed by the DNA. The journey began in the early 1990's, when the author's Tai chi teacher, the miraculous Dr. Marshall Ho'o, mentioned the I-Ching as one of the pillars of Tai Chi Chuan.

VOLUMES TWO AND THREE: ACTIVATION AND COMPLETION

"Activation" is the dynamic process of evolving ideas in the mind to transform our lives and integrate spirit.

To aid in this process, we have an exceptional tool in the art of Tai Chi Chuan. Though it is the principles underlying Tai Chi Chuan that will be our focus, we delve into the details of the form, as well as details on performance, lineage, and philosophy.

In truth, each movement of the Tai chi form is a key that unlocks a part of our genetic encoding, allows us to evolve to our fullest potential. Underlying this art form are principles that, when applied to other areas of life, have a liberating, enhancing effect. This is due to their universality; and due that in the process of their unfoldment, we do not approach consciousness directly.

We "train the mind to train the body." This is much the same as learning anything—how to dance, for instance, or draw, or play a musical instrument. The result is that the mind is *already trained*. We do not have to think about it anymore, we "just do it." Is not this non-reflective, pure state of mind what we are seeking to begin with, as far as the mind is concerned. That we can now do

Tai Chi or play the bassoon, or have increased circulation in the body is just a by-product

Without activation, any spiritual teaching, any philosophy is no better than a pile of paper with ink. Our learning be more than just ideas; it requires the transformation of individual consciousness that comes with the *activation* of those ideas. Meditation, training the mind, mental focus—these things are a life's work at the very least. A constant struggle?

This is why we may consider learning a martial art—to learn how *not* to fight. However, Kung-Fu—which means literally "hard work over a long period of time"—is not the only method of activation. We can also consider the principle of "pilgrimage." This is a journey to a place, a person or an idea—an alignment with principles or a tradition, or with a person.

A pilgrimage allows us direct contact with an energy or energies that somehow changes our perceptions, our focus; some would say it changes our DNA. It can take the form of a visit to a sacred space. There are places on the earth that are so special, they have been pilgrimage spots for longer than recorded history. A pilgrimage can also take the form of meeting with a person;

some feel going to see the Pope or a Tibetan lama at a live appearance has a great effect on the psyche—just being in that person's presence, something is transmitted. The same can be said for conventions of like-minded individuals. If, for example, we were to have a gathering of enough musicians, or chemists, or plumbers—because musicians and chemists and plumbers almost always learn from other musicians, chemists or plumbers—were we to trace the lineage of each individual back far enough, we would have in the room every master who ever lived.

Universality –Volume Three: <u>Completion</u>

This concept of *pilgrimage* has a devotional aspect—the self merging into the large Ocean of Consciousness; as such, it connects with the idea of integration or COMPLETION, which is discussed in our final volume of "White Cloud Journey." Playing Tai Chi or engaging in any creative act that embraces and includes one's entire being— what we call *art*—COMPLETES the energy that created us. The circle that is completed is the circle of life itself.

Some ancient languages, the Tewa language for example, do not have a word for art; the activity was not separated from any other activity. We must assume that the lack of consciousness that made things not an art was not really part of their culture. If the word "beauty" is in the language, then we could make a verb out of that noun; but again, awareness of beauty implies allowing non-beauty into our lives and culture.

The existence of exceptional states—the so-called religious experience or "out-of-body" experience is common to all cultures. However, it is more accurate to call them "in-body experiences"—the body being the infinite realm that expresses the totality of what we are; at the very least, we should include the Earth as part of our body.

Art Forms

Art, whether we have a name for it or not, is the Journey's Return; because a journey in this sense is not just a journey *to* somewhere; it is incomplete without returning. In Islamic tradition, we have the *Ta'wil* (return); it is what makes a metaphor "work"; it is what makes a parable connect with life; it is the punch line to the joke.

Storytelling—the hero's journey, the nature and the principles of art—all of these can be integrated into our daily lives in such a way as to improve the experience for ourselves and others. Yet, there is more to it—

there is a transcendent quality, also a mystery of where it possibly may come from.

We say that a work of art (or a religion or philosophy or a soft drink) is *universal*– meaning, it is useful or comfortable in many different situations, times and places, and for many different people and kinds of people. Another way of comprehending this is tuning in to the holographic nature of our world: taking a small bite off the corner of reality, we find it contains the flavor (informational nexus) of the whole universe.

Yet another way of perceiving this paradigm is *energetic*. We carry the energy of those forces that created us. Allowing those energies to resonate in our creations carries those same "creative" energies forward. The completion of the circle can take place within the individual or between two beings, within a group, or as energy transmitted by way of a work of art. This "thing that happens," this fleeting, momentary experience, is who and what we really are, not what we may seem to be.

The Impersonal Personal

The ancient martial art form of Tai Chi Chuan is a *personal* art form; more exactly, intra-personal; it is used to communicate within one's own personal universe of body/mind/spirit. Meditation in general is such an intra-personal art form. In the following volume of this work, we discuss these arts in more detail, as well as the *inter*-personal art forms of music, painting, cooking, etc. and the medical arts. Those latter forms connect people with one another. However, they have an intra-personal aspect as well; they create for the practitioner an inner life that in some cases transcends earthly limitations. Likewise, Kung-fu (martial arts) is both intra-personal and interpersonal. They first affect the self, but then extend the effect to others.

The Creative Imagination

The Creative Imagination is *first* a mode of perception. It is a way of perceiving truth. This truth is not an intellectual matter; it is determined by the *connection* of the mind/body/universe. If, for instance, we see the light in a person's eyes, or in our own, we can sense—not judge, but *know*— if that light is a true light. We can test its resonance with our totality. If cut off from that totality, then it is a distortion—worse than a lie, it creates the dance of evil. This dance is a solo dance—it only pretends to dance with others.

We cannot approach the development of the creative imagination directly. Rather, it is the part of learning we get from our teachers that comes from their lives: how their lives touch us and not from what they say or even do. Even that is only indirect, because the energy of the Creative Imagination comes *solely* from within the self.

We can only inspire others, not give them the fire of creation. The creative imagination is a form of self-activation; though unpredictable, its development is the subject of Volume Three of this book. The creative imagination is responsible for the return of the self *to* the self, the culmination of the White Cloud Journey.

A NOTE TO THE READER

All we have is time.

We learn that from our elders. Even if we are not inclined to listen to our elders, their lives and especially their deaths invite our attention to the value of time.

If one is fortunate enough to watch someone get old and leave their physical body, one experiences the illusion of standing still and watching time pass by; whereas the reality is much different. The reality is that we are all moving—and extremely fast.

Tai Chi Chuan, "the Art of Living," seems like a long and arduous undertaking—a life-long task to which very few of us may wish to dedicate our lives. Learning Tai Chi requires *slowing way down*. This may not be possible. We may not have a teacher; we may be on a different path, deeply involved in other disciplines; we may be on a fast train going the other direction.

Yet, we can all learn from the vast pool of knowledge that is Tai Chi. In a sense, we all do Tai Chi, whether or not we have even heard the word. Its underlying principles are so universal, so dramatically applicable to every day life that I have never hesitated to recommend this study to anyone, regardless of age, health, ability or whether interested in learning the form, or not.

These same Tai Chi principles can be found in everything and anything. As a Tai Chi activist, I do my best to interest everyone in the form and substance of what I think Tai Chi is. Yet the longer I do so, the more it becomes indistinguishable from anything and everything else—the more I see its truth expressed outside of what anyone would consider Tai Chi. For me, that is the journey: from form to formlessness—the White Cloud Journey.

So, this book is for anyone who wants to know more about Tai Chi, but also for those who want to know about the Tai Chi-ness of the world and themselves.

Jeffrey Fisher

Casablanca, Morocco

March 19, 2009

Contents

Part V: Tai Chi Chuan

As Activation Mode

Part VI. Lifting the Veil

PART FIVE. TAI CHI CHUAN AS AN ACTIVATION CHANNEL

Chapter 14. Keeping Still, Mountain

Tai Chi and I-Ching

Dr. Ho'o spoke of the I-Ching as being the third pillar of Tai Chi Chuan. The Tai Chi Classics mention "...the Five Elements in the feet and the Eight Trigrams in the hands." There have been books (notably, Da Lu) written on the subject of Tai Chi and the I-Ching. However, there is only one reference in the I-Ching itself to "directions for the practice of a Yoga."

The Hexagram KEEPING STILL/MOUNTAIN has "the male principle at the top, striving upward," and the "female principle at the bottom, sinking into the earth." This leaves room in the center for the principles of stillness and relaxation. Relaxing the Kwa, the area between the groin and the legs which connects the lower and upper body, is central to Tai Chi's principles of movement. Tai Chi students will recognize this basic description of a proper Tai

Chi stance: Head suspended; rooted in the earth at all times; Kwa relaxed.

Richard Wilhelm, famed scholar and editor of the I-Ching, remarks that it is significant that the I-Ching, in discussing this Hexagram, speaks of "keeping the back still." The back is the part of the body that one does not see; therefore, it can correspond to the self. When one keeps the self still, one is no longer focusing on the personality or ego.

"Going into his courtyard and not seeing his people," reveals a shift in consciousness: no longer perceiving the self as having an existence separate from the rest of reality.

The *Image* states that the mountains are standing close together—the image of keeping still, the superior man not permitting his thoughts to go beyond his situation. *"Movement has come to its normal end."*

Thus, according to Wilhelm, we have directions for a yoga, meaning *union*, or *joining*. In the previous volume, we discussed semantics and the process of abstraction; how the Chinese language proceeds from the concrete to the abstract. The word *taichi* means *ridgepole,* like the ridgepole that runs down the center of the roof of a house. The purpose of the ridgepole is to connect the two sides; therefore, taichi is anything that *connects polar opposites*—like connecting Yin and Yang.

Therefore, the word Tai Chi—like Yoga—means *union,* or *joining.* Yoga also refers to union of the mind with an energy beyond a definition limited by space and time, as also does Tai Chi Chuan. The tenets of experiential philosophy, as we shall see in the next chapter (Interlude: the Perennial Philosophy), indicate that what we perceive as intelligence is only borrowed intelligence, what we perceive as the self is only the image of the self. Reaching true reality requires a shift in consciousness such as is described in this chapter of the I-Ching, KEEPING STILL/MOUNTAIN.

Life enhancement

Many philosophies and religions are in agreement about stating that the world is illusion (*maya* > mother, matter), that the self is illusion, even that life is illusion. It is not that these things do not exist, but that our perception is distorted. Our limited knowledge, conditioning and concepts places us—in the worst scenario—in a three-dimensional world, bound by time and five senses, living separate existences in physical bodies. Paradoxically, it is only the infinite and universal mind that would be able to cut us off and isolate us in that manner. The more cut off we are, the more active and distorted is our unconscious and subconscious world, the more violent and distorted our social structures become.

Post-Classical Western philosophies have progressed from religion to reason to political ideology to psychology, and we are still faced with the prospect of having to re-create ourselves while we wait for the reconvening of science and religions, long having been separated, possibly by the self-interest of governing bodies.

The physical universe, still a convenient reference point for certain lines of thought and calculation, is now thought by current scientific theory to be a misleading allegory. Science is coming to be closely aligned with the philosophy of Taoism, which for thousands of years has described the universe and its workings in terms of *energy*.

This Taoist "science" is encapsulated in the concepts of Yin and Yang and the theory of the Five Elements, or Five Transformations, which are discussed in the following chapters.

Chapter 15. Tai Chi Chuan and the Perennial Philosophy

An Introduction to Life

Tai Chi Chuan is not per se a philosophy, no less a religion, but for those who practice religiously; yet it is an enhancer and activator of both. Though based on ideas inherent in Taoism, Confucianism and Buddhism, and arising out of that worldview, Tai Chi is primarily a method of training the mind and body. It can help us to live better, think better, and to live our ideas, or to activate those ideas that are at the core of our existence.

The Perennial Philosophy is the title of a short essay by Aldous Huxley that was originally an introduction to Christopher Isherwood's 1929 translation of the Bhagavad-Gita. It is a very clear and complete explanation of the common denominators to the world's major spiritual traditions. The Perennial Philosophy has four main points, as discussed by Huxley, loosely paraphrased here:

1. That the visible universe is but a manifestation of a spiritual realm, without which it would not exist.

2. That all men have a nature that transcends this universe, being part of a larger consciousness.
3. That all men have the ability to access this consciousness intuitively and directly, not merely rationally.
4. That, if life has any importance or meaning, it is in merging the individual self with the larger consciousness.

This is a highest common ground, not a lowest common denominator. It is not a dogma, but a philosophy based on experience rather than ideas. We might conclude that experiential philosophers can take different forms: those like Thoreau, Alan Watts, or Ibn Arabi, whose thoughts usually ran counter to the dogma of their age; people like Jesus, Gandhi, or Martin Luther King, Jr., who actually *lived* their philosophies, whose lives were their testament and gift to the world. We can add yet another category that would include artist and writers, people like Gauguin, Van Gogh, Beethoven, Dostoyevsky, Rumi, Whitman—artists who use an artistic medium to transform souls.

Activating the Energy

However, we must also consider the principle of *activation.* Without activation, any spiritual teaching, any philosophy is no better than a pile of paper with ink. Mohammed described the philosopher who did not live his philosophy as no better than a donkey carrying a load of books. The question, though, is *how?* We are told simply that it is not easy (a camel going through the eye of a needle). We are told to love our neighbor as ourselves, to turn the other cheek, to do unto others, etc. The skill required to do these things is not something we are born with or acquire easily, or learn at school or even the highest university. There have been too few Gandhis, too few Martin Luther King, Jrs. For most of us, successfully turning the other cheek, without succumbing to harm, requires that our learning be more than just ideas; it requires the transformation of individual consciousness that comes with the *activation* of those ideas.

Pilgrimage and Mental Kung-Fu

There are two basic forms of activation: one is the practice in some religions of *pilgrimage.* A pilgrimage allows us direct contact with an energy or energies of a place or a person. This somehow changes our perceptions, our focus; some would say it changes our DNA. These pilgrimages can take different forms. There are the sacred spaces:

places on the earth that are so special, they have been pilgrimage spots for longer than recorded history. (The great Cathedral at Chartres with its famous labyrinth was a pilgrimage spot long before there was a cathedral there.) A pilgrimage can also take the form of meeting with a person; some feel going to see the Pope or a Tibetan lama at a live appearance has a great effect on the psyche—just being in that person's presence, something is transmitted. The same can be said for conventions of like-minded individuals. If, for example, we were to have a gathering of enough musicians—because musicians almost always learn from other musicians—were we to trace the lineage of each musician back far enough, we would have in the room every master who ever lived.

The other form of activation is Kung-Fu, which we already know means hard work over a long period of time; this involves a program for mental training. Usually, mental training takes the form of physical training. Training the mind directly is like building a bridge in the middle of a rushing river, or like psychoanalytic therapy. *However*, if we train the mind to train the body, we find in the end that the mind *is already trained*. As there is really no such thing as physical training that does not include mental training, just about anything done with conscious intent is valuable. This includes any art, whether it is learning a musical instrument, a sport, knitting, splitting firewood, cooking, Yoga, sitting meditation or Tai Chi. The following chapters indicate my bias toward Tai Chi. This is because anyone and everyone is capable of doing it in one form or another; because it enhances health in a number of ways; is inexpensive, requiring no special space, uniform or equipment. Tai Chi, which teaches us how to fight without fighting, can improve just about everything else we do in our lives.

Chapter 16. The Lineage of Tai Chi Masters

The Old and the New

In a dream that recurred or that I dreamed recurred, I am trapped in a large, grey city far to the north. This part of town is deserted, devoid of all life. Even the pigeons are gone. It is bitterly cold, yet I do not feel it as a physical sensation because there seems to be no air to carry the cold. The buildings are old, yet lacking any character; the streets are dirty, the windows soot-covered. There are no cars, no busses. The single road out of town leads only one way: farther to the north—to an endless wilderness of ice and cold.

This image came to mind as I drove over snowpacked roads, over hundreds of miles of frozen wasteland on my way to Montana to do a workshop. I remember that it had been advertised in the area as a "new system of Tai Chi," which was not accurate at all. However, there was some fear out there that the old system would not draw many people.

Americans, especially, seem impressed by the new, the innovative. For some reason, it seems more valuable than mastering something like Tai chi, which is a growing body of knowledge that has been around for hundreds, perhaps thousands of years. This is in sharp contrast to the Chinese tradition, which has as its corresponding weakness a abhorrence of originality and even *development* of traditional ideas.

There is in fact an unbroken lineage of teachers that goes back from Dr. Ho'o to the Thirteenth Century, when a Shaolin priest, Chang San-Feng created a form out of the Kung Fu practiced at the time, the philosophy of the I-Ching, and extensive knowledge of the acupuncture system.

Beginnings

The Kung Fu of Chang's time had been developed seven hundred years previously by Ta Mo, AKA Bodhidharma (see next chapter). He came to the Shaolin monastery from India, probably by way of Tibet, in 527 AD. Finding the monks unhealthy, unable to mediate for long periods, he taught them a series of exercises and training that was so successful that the monks were then able to defend themselves and their community.

The Buddhist monasteries became the source for not only the "hard" (external) schools of martial arts and the "soft" (internal) schools, but for a lot of great Kung Fu movies.

Following Ta Mo's innovations, the monks practiced and developed various exercises and fighting forms; but it was Chang San Feng who is credited with the creation of Tai Chi. His mind was opened when he saw a fight between a snake and a bird. The bird attacked in hard, straight lines, while the snake used circular movements to wear out and overcome the bird. Chang incorporated his knowledge of medicine and healing and philosophy going back to the Yellow Emperor's Book of Internal Medicine (2500 BC), the acupuncture system (which may be as old as 13000 years), and the philosophy of the I-Ching.

This integrated form he taught to a member of the Chen family, where the practice developed in isolation within the family until the 1800's, when Yang Lew Shan brought it into the Yang family and eventually into the rest of China. There were of course as many variations as there were teachers, but the main branch of the Yang Style that has come down to us today is through Yang Chen Fu, who died in 1936.

Marshall Ho'o studied under four of Yang Chen Fu's students: Wen Shan Huang (by way of Tung Ying-Chieh), Chen Wei Ming, Tung Ying Chieh and Yang Zheng Dou; he is thus considered America's first Grandmaster of Yang Style Tai Chi Chuan. With Wen Shan Huang, he started the National Tai Chi Chuan Association. Professor Huang was a well-known author, sociologist, anthropologist and editor. Among his writings are:

SYSTEM OF CULTUROLOGY, 1968

ESSAYS ON CULTURE, 1972

FUNDAMENTALS OF TAI CHI CHUAN, 1973

Translations of:

Bertrand Russell's PROBLEMS OF PHILOSOPHY & ROADS TO FREEDOM

Pitrim Sorokin's CONTEMPORARY SOCIOLOGICAL THEORIES

Joseph Needham's SCIENCE AND CIVILIZATION IN CHINA.

Professor Huang was Department Head of Sociology at National University of Shanghai, Dean of the Law School at National Sun Yat-Sun University, President of Chien Shek University of Shanghai, on the faculty of the New School for Social Research, NYC,

University of Southern California and Columbia University.

He received Tai Chi instruction from great masters all over China as well as studying philosophy in the 1920's with Bertrand Russell and Dr. Hu Shih and obtaining a masters degree from Columbia University. His studies with Tung Ying-Chieh, the eminent pupil of Yang Cheng-fu, made him an outstanding lineage-bearer for the Yang Style of Tai Chi Chuan.

With Marshall Ho'o, he created the longest running Tai Chi class on the West Coast (over 50 years in Bronson Park, LA), and the National Tai Chi Chuan Association, based in Los Angeles.

Yang Style Tai Chi Lineage, the importance of

Many teachers of martial arts, once they have mastered their form to their satisfaction, have gone on to create and teach an altered style, perhaps finding this easier to teach and to learn. After all, Tai Chi has undergone many changes over the past several hundred years, and there have been many valid offshoots from the original Chen style. In fact, no two masters perform the set in exactly the same manner. So why not change the set, give it another name (copyrighted?) and make it more palatable to, for instance, a TV audience who only has ten minutes a week to spare? Wouldn't that reach more people?

This is a valid point. Tai Chi takes more time, commitment, hard work and understanding than most people believe they have to give. Yang Chen-Fu changed the original form to make it easier and more popular. Some say he watered it down so he would not have to teach the Manchu rulers (foreign devils) the real fighting form learned from the Chen family. The original Chen style was extremely acrobatic and took many years to learn, and Yang wanted "everyone" to benefit from Tai Chi. And he was right— today there are probably more Chinese doing Tai Chi on a regular basis than the entire population of the United States. The legendary Chen Man-Ch'ing created his "short form" for the same reason; he was teaching classes to the army and needed a form that was faster and easier to learn.

The plethora of Tai Chi styles and even vast differences within the Yang Style can be confusing to the novice. Students sometimes slavishly copy the form of their teachers and then pass it on to their students without considering whether it is correct, or whether differences with other styles are improvements or defects. A style of a particular master may change greatly with time and state of health; or he or she may teach people with different abilities and needs slightly or distinctly different forms.

There are valid reasons not to change the form. Tai Chi is more than an exercise—it is a philosophy and a way of life, and a link with many branches of philosophy (actually, with the whole of Chinese culture going back at least 5,000 years). It is a *direct* link with all the teachers of the past, going back to Chang

San-Feng in the 1200's. Recently, there has been tremendous research and input by Western teachers, and it's all contained in the form. In other words the form itself is a living entity—it records changes, and the vision and energy of all who have ever or ever will "play Tai Chi." Changing the form entails a huge responsibility.

A good teacher gives a great deal of himself—to the art, and to those he teaches. This gives a personal aspect to the experience of learning which is more important than any hierarchy of "who studied with whom." Authenticity of teaching is something felt, anyway; Tai Chi is not learned from a book, videotape, or even from another person. A teacher can only mirror and point the way.

Tai Chi is something that must be experienced. There is an inner teaching that occurs, a universal force that is neither the energy of the teacher nor of the student, but part of what is termed the "Tai Chi space." One enters this is a space when undertaking the discipline of learning the form. The time and work involved in learning the complexities of the form is amply rewarded. What gives Tai Chi it's amazing curative and regenerative power is the involvement and commitment of the practitioner.

Certainly the form may be altered to accommodate a physical problem or for instructing beginners of a certain age group. However, constructing something new out of the elements that seem most beneficial is akin to removing or synthesizing the "active ingredients" of a medicinal herb used for centuries in its whole form. Who knows what is really in the plant that may be there to balance, to instruct, to catalyze? Who knows what Tai Chi is, what its origins were, and what its connections are to the human body and the universe.

Chapter 17. The Purpose of Tai Chi Chuan

Ta-Mo and Buddhist Teaching

Tai Chi Chuan is an effective and powerful martial art. Traditionally (in *Tai Chi* tradition, of course), Tai Chi masters have succeeded in vanquishing opponents from all other martial arts forms. Even more powerful is its potential for healing and maintaining health, though this aspect is still a young science in this country. Examining history, a figure emerges who may expand our concept of the purpose and meaning of the art of Tai Chi Chuan.

In 528 A.D. the Buddhist monk Ta-Mo arrived from India arrived at the Shao-lin monastery. Finding the devotees engrossed in the spiritual and mental aspects of Buddhism but too physically weak to maintain concentration for long periods of time, he instituted a series of exercises that eventually developed into the various forms of *kung-fu*, or martial arts.

Records suggest he is only the second major teacher of Buddhism to arrive from India in the 500 years since the establishment of Buddhism in India. The possible significance of this fact is that the Chinese practitioners of those years relied on texts or *interpretation of texts by those who could read them*; they lacked a more balanced approach, including physical training, which could be transmitted only by personal instruction. Compare the Buddhism of Tibet, which includes many aspects of physical training, with Chinese Buddhism, which relied on written material in an era when "secrets" were rarely written (or so well hidden that they were not revealed for hundreds of years); they may have lost much of these teachings until the time of Ta-Mo.

The works of Ta-Mo include "The Muscle and Tendon Changing Classic" and the "Brain and Marrow Washing Classic". These books include instructions for circulating and developing energy (*chi*) and using this energy to strengthen and maintain the body and mind. Did this information originally come from India or was it a synthesis of what already existed in Chinese Taoism, which seems to emphasize more in the realm of health? Was it totally original work, or did Ta-Mo incorporated something he learned elsewhere, such as in Tibet?

Ta Mo's Classics were not designed to increase martial skills or even to increase health for its own sake, but to help the practitioner achieve Enlightenment, a state of oneness with the truth of our existence which may prevent rebirth into suffering and ignorance.

Ta-Mo, often referred to as Bodhidharma, is an important link in the chain of Tai Chi forerunners, and surprisingly, is also the patriarch of Karate. His work shows us that Tai Chi practice need not be limited to physical training and that physical training has a definite place in our spiritual development.

Chapter 18.
Karma and Tai Chi

Our current understanding of karma is that it is a natural law--*everything that occurs affects the universe as a whole.* Thus, when one acts, or speaks, or thinks, one makes changes that affect everything, including oneself.

Just as a strong wind might bend a tree, or remove a roof from a house, yet be stopped by a mountain, forces in the universe are relative to one another: stronger energies may absorb and repulse the weaker. Since the physicality of the universe grasps our attention at an early age, we take for granted this connection of energy.

The other aspect of karma, that every action we perform comes back to us, seems more far-fetched. This is because of the density of matter in our three-dimensional universe. On subtler planes of existence, just thinking a harmful thought may cause harm; the denseness of our physical plane protects us to a certain extent.

As to the actual *mechanism* of karma, one theory is that vibration within our genetic encodement is responsible for much that is beyond our conscious thought. The DNA itself (and supposedly, the *vibratory rate* of our DNA is what separates us from other beings) records everything that occurs. Its crystalline structure is capable of transmitting energy as well, and it is likely that information is transmitted and encoded in the fabric of the universe itself. Nothing that happens in life is ever lost.

Because Tai Chi mirrors, harmonizes and resonates with the "vortex energy" of genetic material, doing the form can put us in touch with parts of ourselves that are hidden or enfolded in the DNA itself. We can change or restructure our lives—past, present and future—and come to a greater understanding of our potential as humans. We are not looking to find within this exercise a mathematical correlation such as we find in music; we are simply acting with intent, yet without expectation or attachment to results.

We might liken this to prayer (without theology), or meditation (without the mind). At the same time, we can see karma as the structure of the divine path of light. This structure allows for the self-correcting functioning and evolution of consciousness in the universe. There is no difference between evolution (physical) and spiritual growth, if we are all part of God and part of the Divine

Plan. We can visualize this as inter-dimensional six-sided bits of information, functioning as holographic film around the evolutionary spiral of DNA. This is acti-vated by the vibrational nature of conscious-ness— our own consciousness and that of other living beings with whom we come in contact.

God cannot be perceived as a separate being, just as we cannot perceive ourselves as a separate being, since we are inside ourselves and inside God. Holography requires at least two coherent light sources for projec-tion to take place. Our own conscious emanation causes the reflection that creates our perception of the "universe."

The amino acid structure that comprises the DNA has been described as combinations of the 6-bit pattern--totaling 64 different com-binations, like the I-Ching. The activation of the combinations, due to the condensed nature of these structures, depends upon the frequency of the vibrational ray that pene-trates. The higher the vibraional rate, the greater the activation.

How does this crystalline structure of the DNA store "karmic" information? Why do trees, each whose seed may come from the same pinecone and may appear identical, grow into a different size and shape? One piece may turn out to be firewood, the other a Stradivarius. The question "why?" is its own answer.

Is the concept of karma different from that of sin? If we are punished or rewarded in the next life or an afterlife, is that a difference? In reality, there is neither afterlife nor a "next" life, but the patterns persist, outside of time, and life continues infinitely. We are expressions of these infinite patterns. What lives, dies. But what "we" are cannot die, nor can it really live in the sense of "what lives, dies." We are beyond that, and beyond matter except as the gift of experience allows us to work through the plane of matter either for our own benefit or the benefit of other parts of the whole. (And the concept of "benefit" is also dubious, since our concept of "purpose" is limited to what we see here, and what we see here cannot be said to have a "purpose." Yet the concept "purpose" has to have come from somewhere, so we can say that *we* might have a purpose here, even though life itself may not.)

From an acquaintance, a writer who may or may not have ever written this down, comes the story of a visit to an isolated monastery, in the vaults of which are hidden one of the two remaining copies of the original New Testament (the other sequestered in the Vati-

Vatican). The translation of the text reveals the word "repent" to be the same term used by ancient horsemen to turn their animals 180 degrees. For years after he told me this story I interpreted it to mean that we repentance has less to do with confession of sin and prayer than changing our lives in a more "positive" direction.

That is undoubtedly part of the interpretation. But what of the sin itself? What of the implications of traveling in the "wrong" direction? Can that sin or karma can be wiped out the moment we turn from it? The economical quality of the ecology of the universe would indicate that moment we change directions, we correct our mistake, and we do not have to carry our corrections along with us. Death is part of life and the greatest gift to life. But our own gift to ourselves is the ability to erase our mistakes and not carry around guilt, the root of all other addictions.

Chapter 19.

Relaxation & Wu-Wei

--The Power of Not-Doing

Doing Nothing is Easy

Wu-wei , a Taoist term meaning ^*not doing*, is sometimes associated with a heightened state of awareness and acts bordering on magical. However, we can find a concrete basis for *wu-wei* in the simple act of relaxing.

Relaxation is a state if being that requires release of tension—tension being energy, but not necessarily energy that can be utilized efficiently. In Tai Chi practice, the Chinese word *sung* is associated with a state "relaxed attention," or hyper-awareness coupled with lack of unnecessary tension.

If at first we may think of "relaxed attention" as a paradox, or even an oxymoron, we can change our thinking. Instead of presuming relaxation to be good, and tension as bad, we can see tension and release in a yin and yang sort of balance, with each taking up half the space, and *sung* being the dynamic balance of tension and release. Realizing that tension is *energy*, we can be more efficient, even effortless in our movements.

How to Relax without Really Trying

Sung is a physical and mental/emotional state that borders on a mystical experience; but in Tai Chi, we first approach *sung* through the body, relaxing all the muscles not needed to perform a specific movement. We also control the breath, making sure that it is deep, natural and even. This increases the flow of chi, or vital energy throughout the body, as well the flow of blood, oxygen and lymph.

Since all tension manifests in the body, it would be reasonable to surmise that all we would need to deal with tension skillfully would be to pay attention to the body. However, our definition of the body had better be inclusive: since there is no definite division between the body and the mind, or the emotional, spiritual, astral and energetic aspects, the body really includes all that we are. And since all that we are is defined by all that we are not, we must pay attention to *everything.* This is really simpler and easier than having to decide where to place our attention, especially since those types of decisions are usually conditioned responses and not so intelligent as our natural, centered response coupled with the 70% Rule. (The 70% Rule, for those unfamiliar with Tai Chi practice, basically means not putting all your eggs in one basket.)

Sticking to it

Besides having a definition of the self that extends to infinity, it helps to look inward and perceive an infinite inward space as well; then, to have a strategy for dealing with what we find there. This is also easy, because we use the same strategy we use on what is "outside." We neither grasp nor attempt to block or push away these energies, be it an enemy, a stray thought, or an emotion. We merely pay attention, welcome, perhaps even bow (without lowering our eyes).

Just as in push-hands, we stick to our opponent, *following* the energy. Yang always changes to yin; an aggressive force always wears itself out. By sticking, harmonizing with the energy instead of fighting it, an attack becomes a "gift," a potentially obsessive thought or emotion becomes merely extra motivation. This is the core of relaxation, of *sung* and of Tai Chi training, and our particular way of approaching Wu-Wei, or *not-doing.*

Chapter 20.

The Five Aspects and the Twenty-Five Benefits of Tai Chi

One could divide the study and practice of Tai Chi into five somewhat overlapping aspects. The first is that of health. The various positive effects and cures are discussed elsewhere in this book, but exactly why does it work?

Slow, gently stretching movements, correct posture and alignment combined with relaxation increase the flow of energy through the acupuncture meridians to all parts of the body. Health and healing are aided by the slowing down of breathing and brain waves.

Tai Chi is also a superior form of exercise for the reason that it allows a wide scope of interest and depth of involvement. Any exercise is only as good as the person doing it--i.e., it's hard to get anything out of something you're not doing.

Complementary to the health aspect is that of martial arts, which is both art and science. It is an extension and refinement of the health aspect, teaching us how to perceive and use energy, in the world and within oneself. The paradox is that though we start by learning a form, the goal is spontaneity--free expression of energy.

As martial arts training progresses from form to formlessness, from limitation of the physical to transcendence, from conditioned responses to accurate perception of reality, we are led to the spiritual aspect of Tai Chi. In some ways, this aspect is a combination of health and martial arts--as, for instance, in the focusing and sending out of healing energies. In the context of Tai Chi, one could define spirituality as the practice of self-knowledge and the experience of unity.

This is obviously a big subject, and most people have their own interpretations of what is spiritual. Why is Tai Chi any more spiritual that playing baseball or the stock-market? Tai Chi may be more universal, and therefore more practical as a way of life. Again, one can be only as spiritual as one's ability to practice that spirituality. It must be stressed that Tai Chi is not a religion; i.e., it gives us no set way for dealing with the spiritual aspect of our lives. It is an enhancer of any path that we have chosen.

This brings us to the fourth aspect: that of ritual. A ritual is any activity, done on a regular basis, which connects us to our "larger" or "higher" existence. The cycle of rituals of the Catholic Church, for instance, connects us to the life of Jesus. Something as mundane as brushing our teeth can connect us to a higher principle of self-care based on self-awareness. Doing the 108 regularly can put one in touch with one's basic physical-mental-emotional-spiritual-earthly energies—for better health, greater productivity, more harmonious relationships, or just a more pleasant day. Combining the other three aspects, it is ritual that joins us to others that are practicing. Even though the art is personal, the journey and the experience can be shared.

Tai Chi also has a symbolic aspect. By extending our range of motion by imitating animal movement, we recognize our commonality and connection with all lifeforms. The totality of the form, beginning to end, also symbolizes or is a metaphor of one's whole life, birth to death, and the whole evolution of life—darkness to light.

Benefits—Please Read Carefully

The benefits of doing Tai Chi depend upon the individual--his or her abilities, interest and focus. Learning is therefore a non-competitive situation. Very briefly, Tai Chi has benefits in the following areas:

PHYSICAL EXERCISE

1. stretches the muscles and tendons, promotes flexibility

2. aerobically stimulates (brings oxygen to) muscles, tendons, organs,
3. bones and bone marrow
4. exercises (gently) the heart and lungs; do-able by persons of any age or physical condition.
5. (large circles) strengthen legs and large muscle groups
6. (small circles) stimulate organs and endocrine function
7. improves coordination by connecting lower and upper body
8. promotes circulation of blood (stretching veins, arteries and capillaries; thus, making the heart's work easier).
9. Promotes circulation of lymph (by focusing on fold and unfold of Kwa).
10. helps posture and alignment, thus relieving backaches, pinched nerves or other symptomatic results of stress
11. balances energy and organ systems

12. stimulates meridian system, resulting in improved immune system; balances body chemistry
13. helps balance, rejuvenate, regenerate entire body and mind

MEDITATION

14. by slowing the body movements and slowing the breath, the mind is slowed to the point of being able to control thoughts
15. balance of mind and body, focus of intent
16. learning the philosophy of Yin and Yang, learning the "middle way," avoiding extremes
17. "rooting" (using gravity and the forces of nature to our benefit rather than being in conflict)
18. "circulation of chi": learning to heal ourselves and others through the use of the energy within and around us
19. learning the philosophies of Buddhism, Taoism, Confucianism and the I-Ching tend to promote mental and emotional health and well-being.
20. movements seen as body-mudras/movement mantras, extend-

ing heart/mind ritualistically through higher planes of self-awareness

MARTIAL ARTS

21. learning the real meaning of kung-fu
22. using "four ounces to deflect 1000 pounds"
23. "push hands" practice: sensitivity to another's energy and intent
24. transforming self, conquering space, time, reality
25. maintaining non-judgmental emotional environment; becoming unconditional love

Chapter 21. The Five Transformations

Think of the circular motion of a motor. Think of the circular motion of the earth, shifting from night to day. Think of the wave-like pulse of a city, of electricity, sound waves; a heartbeat, or the ocean.

Think of going to a market or a fruit-stand and seeing an apple. The apple may not speak to you in words, but it has an energy that communicates to your body, energy that merges with your mind before you (consciously) decide to buy the apple to eat.

Life is an energetic process; understanding the moods or phases of energy is a way to understand life. This is what we call the Five Elements, or sometimes the Five Transformations of Energy. The cycle of Fire, Earth, Metal, Water and Wood underlies much of Chinese philosophy, medicine and martial arts.

The correspondences and differences with the Western Hermetic version of earth, air, fire and water are evident after some study and appreciation of the ancient Chinese system.

Sometimes it is very useful to view everything in our world as solid, even though science and higher intuitive processes say it is not. At other times, being stuck in that vision of the world is not useful, and we do better tuning into the phases of energy. Energy is fluid--it can blend with other energies, or separate at will; it can change and transform. If life is an equation always seeking balance within itself, and if we are seeking within our own lives to evolve and manifest what our inner being envisions, then being able to adjust our concept of solidity vs. energy is very helpful.

For instance, if we allow ourselves to make decisions based on a conditioned view of the world as solid, then we may miss some subtle clue as to the true nature of that reality. Part of Tai Chi training— learning to play with energy—is about letting energies play themselves out, neither grasping, nor pushing away. It is a way to act out of compassion rather than fear; to not be manipulated by events by giving up need to control everything.

The Five Transformations is just another way to understand the workings of energy in our world. For instance, think of Wood transforming itself in a Fire. The upward energy of Fire shifts as the ashes fall back to Earth. The downward direction continues as pressure mounts within the Earth, creating Metal. Deep within the Earth, the pressure is so great that that heat is created and metals melt. This is the energy of Water, liquefying, rising and giving life to Wood; and the cycle continues.

The Five Energies are also the basis of Chinese Traditional Medicine, each element corresponding to a pair of internal organs:

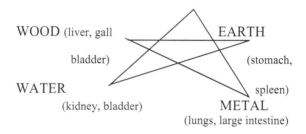

FIRE (heart, small intestine)

WOOD (liver, gall bladder)

EARTH (stomach, spleen)

WATER (kidney, bladder)

METAL (lungs, large intestine)

These Five Transformations express one cycle of energy, from the Yang extreme of Fire to the Yin extreme between Metal and Water. This cycle also correlates to the seasons (the Chinese have five), and to all cycles of energy expressed by the self, the universe and their interaction. They are used in Chinese medicine as a guide to the interaction of the organs and systems of the body. Again, it is sometimes helpful to view these organs and systems more as energetic functions rather than purely anatomical structures.

We can see the energy traveling in two cycles: the Creative and Destructive (or Controlling). We have already discussed the Creative Cycle: Water feeding Wood, Wood feeding Fire, Fire to Earth, Earth to Metal, Metal to Water . The Controlling Cycle is: Earth to Water (earth dams control the flow of water), Water to Fire (water extinguishes fire), Fire to Metal (fire melts metal), Metal to Wood (metal cuts wood), Wood to Earth (roots of trees breaking up earth).

These ideas reflect the rural simplicity of Chinese culture of 5000 years ago, yet they have been very effective for all this time in treatment of disease. For instance, to treat a stomach ailment, it can be helpful to strengthen the lungs (Creative Cycle). To ease the heart (high blood pressure, for example), excess energy (blockage) of the kidneys is relieved, using the Controlling Cycle.

The Tai Chi Classics say to "practice with the eight trigrams (of the I-Ching) in the arms, and the Five Elements under the feet."

The meaning of this is not to be taken lightly, or explained simply. Often, by practicing the movements for a while—which can be several hours or several years—one can come to an understanding of the connection.

The process of taking a step, of putting one foot in front of the other and walking, is simple enough, once we learn it as a child, that we take it for granted. In Tai Chi, however, we slow the process down to examine and learn from the elements involved. For instance, the act of rocking from heel to toe is part of a circle—we invented the wheel as an extension of our feet. We can reverse the process and learn better how to walk by examining the wheel. To achieve a smooth flow of movement from one foot to another, we prepare each movement; we have the heel of the unweighted foot already in place before transferring the weight from the other side. That involves thinking ahead, which is thinking backwards around the circle. (We can even break down some of the movements, such as the "Twisting Step," into five interconnecting sections.) Different ways of moving also activate different energy meridians and help different organs and organ systems.

Ancient Western alchemy, like Taoist alchemy, uses the Elements as basic aspects of consciousness. The goal is transmutation of the baser elements into the finer (lead into gold). The concept of "as above, so below" means that the process works on all levels—material and spiritual. It is interesting that alchemy "developed" into chemistry, which in the early part of the last century arrived at the concept of the identity of matter and energy, and lately re-discovered the transmutation of elements. Evolving spiritually involves developing links between energy levels; consciousness of the Five Elements, like a space ship, links heaven and earth.

PART SIX :

LIFTING THE VEIL—

FORM AND BEYOND

"When the student appears, the teacher is ready."

--JEFFREY FISHER "FRACTURED QUOTES"

Chapter 22. The Best

Insurance is Prevention

- **CONSULT YOUR TAI CHI TEACHER BEFORE GOING TO A DOCTOR.**

- **PROPER WARM-UP BEFORE EXERCISE PREVENTS INJURIES— STRETCHING BEFORE AND AFTER IS ALSO GOOD.**

- **REMEMBER, THE KNEE IS A HINGE JOINT AND NOT MEANT TO BE TORQUED. IT SHOULD ALWAYS STAY IN ALIGNMENT WITH THE TOE AND HIP, AND NEVER BENT MORE THAN OVER THE TOE**

- **TO PROTECT THE KNEES WHEN WORKING ON A CARPET OR OTHER NON-SKID SURFACE, THE MOVEMENTS MIGHT HAVE TO BE SLIGHTLY MODIFIED WHILE TURNING OR PIVOTING. MAKE SURE TO TAKE THE WEIGHT**

OFF THE FOOT THAT'S TURN-
ING.

- ALL THE BODY IS CONNECTED
  WITH THE SPINE. BEFORE
  PRACTICING OR DOING ANY-
  THING STRENUOUS, STOMACH
  ROTATIONS (SEE WARM-UPS)
  ARE ESSENTIAL.

- NEVER FORCE A MOVEMENT OR
  A STRETCH—EVERY TAI CHI
  MOVEMENT CAN BE DONE AT
  ONE'S OWN LEVEL OF COM-
  FORT WITHOUT SACRIFICING
  FORM OR FLUIDITY. STRETCH—
  DON'T STRAIN.

- IN TAI CHI, POWER COMES
  FROM RELAXATION. STRETCH-
  ING IS ALSO RELAXING—
  BREATHE OUT DURING A
  STRETCH.

- DEPARTING FROM THE CENTER,
  ACCIDENTS AND ILLNESS OC-
  CUR. MAINTAIN CENTER
  THROUGH CONSISTENT TAI CHI
  PRACTICE. THIS IS THE TOOL
  THAT HELPS PREVENT AND

AVOID ILLNESS AND ACCI-DENTS.

- **LISTEN TO YOUR BODY, STAY IN TOUCH WITH YOUR ENERGY; ILLNESSES AND ACCIDENTS HAPPEN FIRST IN THE MIND AND THE EMOTIONAL BODY.**

Chapter 23.

Three Non-Lessons

1. Welcome To the Middle Way

Entering the Tai Chi space, enters the self—the body/mind/spirit—not through the front door, but through the service entrance. One is engaged in the process of tuning up, re-adjusting and in fact rewiring all systems.

Though passed down for thousands of years, in various forms, generation to generation, Tai Chi is a personal art form. It is one's own relationship to the practice that is important, not how much one knows or can do compared with someone else.

Usually, there is someone around who knows more, or less, or something different. This makes it possible for us all to help each other to learn.

We all have different and varying abilities. Those with less ability may be able to learn and achieve more in a shorter time; but for everyone, the beginning feels awkward, perhaps frustrated. There seems so much to learn! One is supposed to relax, and it is impossible to relax when first learning. Yet even from that beginning, from the very first movement, one is forming new connecting links between the mind and body.

During the journey, it is common for the ego to inquire whether one's time might be better spent learning something of more practical value, like knitting, or microbiology; or, something more spiritual, like the Bible or Mahayana Buddhism. The fact is, it really does not matter; as we shall see, the truth underlying Tai Chi is the truth underlying all of life.

The fact that you are reading this book means that there is a reason you are exploring Tai Chi. For some it is health, for some it is martial arts training, for others it is a spiritual adventure and a healing art. Regardless, the learning priorities are the same: study the principles, understand the postures, and learn the sequence. The real work is done high on a rocky precipice overlooking a great mountainous valley. Here, one experiences the infiniteness of mind, the boundlessness of the body and the reality that Tai Chi is one thing you can do the rest of your life (if not forever) and luckily never learn it all.

2. *Lesson One*

Tai Chi could be considered the art of movement.

Movement is life, is breath, is vibration, is thought, emotion and communication.

Movement is always relative to something--to ourselves or to the earth. So earth is important, as a reference point; and air, as a medium for movement--something to swim in. The word orientation refers to our cosmic position--the sun (fire element)--which gives us the ten directions that define our world. Left, right, up, down, forward and backward are meaningless without east, west, north, south, earth and sky.

The Five Elements (also known as the Five Energies or Five Transformations: earth, metal, water, wood and fire) can describe the qualities of movement: hard or soft, full or empty---how it flows.

The position of earth and sky, and our connection to them also define the speed of motion. Most Tai Chi movements are relatively slow.

Why is this? To slow down usually means an increase in awareness, in control of movements (the mind controlling the body rather than vice versa). When we slow down, we change breathing and physiology, thinking patterns and psychology as well. When we slow down, we "see" more, and it is easier to achieve perfection of thought and movement and intent.

It is easy to sense the healing potential of such slow movement, but what of the martial arts aspect? Why do practitioners consider Tai Chi the ultimate martial art? Though form and physics are important, and each movement has a martial application, this aspect goes beyond form. There are underlying principles that help one develop the mind, body and spirit to realize unity with all things. Marshall Ho'o is known for the statement: "Tai Chi is the art of living."

3. *Yin and Yang*

YIN & YANG

The Tai Chi symbol

represents Yin and Yang.

The circle appears still, but

is in continuous motion--Yin

becoming Yang, and Yang

becoming Yin, just as the seasons

revolve and energy circulates.

(Motion within stillness is the key to

Tai Chi movement.

Stillness within movement is the key to

listening to the universe.)

At the fullness of each phase, the seed of its opposite appears, Yin and Yang being the two poles, the two basic forms of energy that exist everywhere, from the beginning to the end of the universe. Yin is the dark, contracting, the "negative" force, Yang is the light, expanding, "positive."

These two energies are found in varying, complementary amounts in everything, so that one thing relative to another is always more yin or more yang.

In Tai Chi Chuan, we consider these forces in their most basic, physical and manageable form: full and empty, or weighted and un-weighted. When play with full and empty, when we learn about weighted and un-weighted, we are playing and learning about Yin and Yang, we are experiencing infinity.

Chapter 24. How To Practice

It is said, in many systems of learning, that if a person does a new activity or practices a new skill *consistently for 90-100 days,* it becomes part of that person. Inconsistent practice for twice or three times that period will not produce the commensurate results. At one's first stages of practice, working long hours for many days, then doing nothing is not as effective as doing a little bit every day.

For building strength and endurance, it is good to work the body 20 to 40 minutes, depending on intensity of the workout); this is one reason that the Yang Style Long Form has many repeats and takes so long to perform. However, as in any new activity, it is important to build up slowly.

There is only one real secret to learning a new skill: to do it. Integrating a new activity into an already busy schedule may be a problem. The following steps might be helpful:

(a) **Set a specific time for practice.** Very often, schedules are like cupboards or suitcases: much more can be fit in by rearranging them. At first, it may be necessary to *establish* the time for practice--by getting up ten minutes earlier, for instance.

(b) Making a commitment. *"If not now, when?"* generates superabundant energy, as a person is focused and aligned with the higher self; the universe never fails to respond to the flow by attracting like energies.

(c) **Knowing you can do it.** Know that we are usually attracted to some necessary at first. However, we are usually attracted to things for some deeper reason. *Believing* is not enough, and may not even be necessary. Often, doing the work itself can unite one with one's true nature.

(d) **Keep the big picture in mind.** Anything new can feel good right away; but the feeling diminishes as one falls back to old habits. With Tai Chi exercise, it may take six weeks to show results of any sort. In five years you may have a new body and a new life. In twenty years, you may begin to master the form. *Time itself*--doing something in many different contexts, through many life-changes--can produce miracles by improving confidence.

(e) **Do it all the time.** Make it part of your consciousness. Apply the principles to every thought and every action. An artist or musician feeds his art through the uncon-

scious so that everything that occurs becomes transformed into an expression of the
heart. In the same way, we can *become* Tai
Chi, or anything that we choose to lea

Chapter 25.

Warm-up Exercises

As preliminary to Tai Chi or any other form of

movement, exercise or just

sitting around

Note: These exercise are derived from various sources—some are almost universal Tai Chi warm-ups. They developed in the Buddhist temples with the various styles of kung-fu, or as health and meditation exercises in the Taoist temples; others are from Yoga or dance or other martial arts forms.

It is usually important to incorporate Tai Chi principles into the warm-ups as well as the form. For example, they are all done slowly, with energy sunk, back straight, head suspended. Watch your alignment, be aware of weight shifts, and stay relaxed (especially shoulders and elbows). Rarely does the knee bend farther out than the toes.

The purpose of these exercises is to develop strength and flexibility, but especially to move the energy of the vascular, lymphatic, nervous and meridian systems. That is why they are done in a relaxed manner, with the utmost concentration on the intent of each motion. The principle of reciprocal movement is also very important—if an exercise is done on one side it is then done on the other side. This is to balance the movement; daily activities that consist in repetitive movements on one side only can cause chronic problems.

All of the exercises are helpful for doing the form correctly or better. They are also helpful for a particular physical problem or ailment, and can be done singly, with many repetitions.

1. Stomach rotations

Feet together, knees straight but not locked. Palms of hands on kidneys--rotate the navel forming horizontal circle. Reverse. Concentrating on tan tien, feel the spiraling up of heat-energy. Focus on the circle on the plane parallel to the ground; stop at sore places—breathe through them. Good for loosening the spine, also for digestive organs. Variations: (a) hands at sides, feet slightly wider, knees more bent; good for mid-back

2. Knee rotations

Back straight, feet together, hands on knees, bend knees, drawing horizontal circles, head at constant height (not bobbing). Reverse. Good for spleen, warms up knees to prevent injury, strengthens legs.

3. Picking fruit

Arms raised, shoulders near ears. Feet apart, shoulder width, legs straight. Fold at Kwa, turning slightly and stretch up—one side of the body at a time: fingers, wrist, elbow, shoulder, waist, hips, knees, ankles, feet— opening all joints. Then relax, leaving the arm raised slightly, and do the other side. Variation: put fruit behind back. Loosens up back of neck, shoulders, massages me- ridians of heart, bladder. Good for general energy, blood pressure.

4. Cross-arm swing

Legs straight, shoulder-width, arms ex- tended, spread-eagle, palms forward. Turn at the waist, keeping hips straight forward, clap hands together. Good for flexibility of waist, massages kidney area. Alternate sides.

5. Shoulder rotations

Keeping knees and arms loose, rotate the shoulders, up to the ears, then back down, first one direction, then the opposite. Let whole body move. SI meridian and back of neck.

6. Elbows on knees

Grasping hands together, place bent elbows on knees, and sit down. Straighten up, with back straight. Stretches, strengthens back of legs.

7. Stretching

Bending at waist with back straight, with fingers laced, stretch downwards in small circular movements, first with feet slightly apart, then with heels and toes together.

Think of lengthening muscles. Keep back straight at all times, do not look down, and keep knees straight.

8. Advance/Retreat

In horse-stance (feet shoulder width apart, knees bent), fold on the Kwa, to the right or left, shift weight in that direction, "riding the horse" (not bobbing).

To Retreat, shift weight backwards, then turn. Slowly, arms relaxed, feet parallel. To Advance, first turn, then shift forward.

9. Prayer Wheel

In bow stance (with feet together, turn left foot out at 45degrees, step forward at shoulder's width with right foot), hands in front, about one foot apart, shifting weight from front to back, arms turn in a circle. Continue leg movement, move arms in swimming motion, then gathering in. Repeat on other side.

10. Leg Swings

Turn one foot 45 degrees and swing the other foot off the ground. Feel spine stretch and loosen. Grab foot with opposite or same hand from behind and stretch the leg. Balance and reach down to touch toe. Still standing on one foot, pull the knee up to chest. Then, with knee cocked, open pelvis and stand with arms in "hugging tree" (standing meditation) position. If balance is stable, close eyes. Extend leg as far and high as possible, rotate ankle (each direction five times), then rotate knee and hip, similarly. Grab foot and straighten leg. Good for balance, strengthens leg, loosens spine, also good for organs, immune system.

11. Advanced stretching

Leg extended or up on bar, chair, table or tree; back straight; leg in front straight. Bend from waist to touch head to toe, or as close as possible. On the floor, Splits, with each leg forward, and to side.

12. Neck and Shoulders

Turning head, look to the left, back to center, then to the right. Look up and back in either direction, then down and back, at opposite heel.

13. Neck and Shoulders II

Place right arm over left shoulder.   With crook of left elbow push back on right elbow while turning head as far as possible to the right. Grab the ear lobe with fingers of right hand. Reverse.

14. Grinding Corn

With legs double shoulder width apart, squat down, knees over toes, back straight, arms in front (palms down) in circular motion on the lateral plane. Shift weight from left to right, folding Kwa.

Reverse the circles.

15. Horse Stance

Legs shoulder width, feet parallel, weight sunk, head suspended, back straight. Knees bowed out like riding a horse, and bent slightly, over the toes. Tailbone pointing straight into the earth.

16. Shanghai Hospital Exercise

This exercise stimulates the lung and heart meridians and has been used to help tuberculosis patients. Feet shoulder width, arms in front 30 degrees. Swing arms vigorously back (like getting ready to do a standing broadjump), and let them swing naturally back to the 30 degrees in front.

CHAPTER 26. YANG STYLE SHORT FORM

1. **COMMENCEMENT--S**

2. **PARTING WILD HORSE'S MANE--E**

3. **WHITE STORK COOLS ITS WINGS**

4. **BRUSH KNEE 3 TIMES**

5. **PLAY THE GUITAR**

6. **REPULSE MONKEY 4 TIMES**

7. **GRASP THE BIRD'S TAIL, LEFT SIDE**

8. **TURN, GRASP BIRD'S TAIL, RIGHT SIDE--W**

9. SINGLE WHIP--E

10. WAVE HANDS LIKE CLOUDS, S

11. SINGLE WHIP--E

12. SEPARATE RIGHT FOOT

13. HIT TO EARS,—SE

14. TURN (LEFT) AND KICK LEFT HEEL--W

15. SNAKE CREEPS DOWN, LEFT

16. GOLDEN COCK STANDS ON L. FOOT

17. SNAKE CREEPS DOWN, RIGHT

18. GOLDEN COCK ON R. FOOT

19. FAIR LADY AT THE SHUT-
TLES, R,L (NW &SW)

20. NEEDLE AT SEA BOTTOM

21. FAN THROUGH BACK—
>N>E

22. TURN AND CHOP

23. STEP, PARRY, PUNCH

24. WITHDRAW, PUSH, CROSS
HANDS AND CLOSE--S

Chapter 27. Why do the Long Form?

The way we learn Tai chi is not a straight diagonal line. It is more like a state change. An example of state change is ice melting. The ice absorbs a certain amount of energy before it starts to change. The freezing point of ice is 32 degrees, as is the melting point. After it melts, the water now measures 32 degrees, but a state change has occurs. The same applies to water freezing: it has to maintain the freezing-point temperature for a while before it becomes ice.

At a certain point, we start to pick up—our practice picks up—we are really doing Tai Chi instead of isolated movements. A critical mass is reached. The body and mind are moving in harmony instead of being at odds.

Is the Long Form more conducive to this happening than the Short Form? If so, then why did Marshall Ho'o utilize the Short Form, at least for beginners?

The short form has its advantages: one can get to some of the more interesting and challenging movements without having to tax the brain with memorizing a long sequence. But is it really the brain that is taxed? The Chinese, when thinking or referring to what actually learns always refer to the heart. Even in our culture, when we talk of memorizing something, we say "learn it by heart."

Tai Chi emphasizes the mind being in control. It is said that, "Chi (energy) follows the mind." Dr. Ho'o used to talk of the uselessness of what he called "unmotivated action;" i.e., exercise that does not have the mind engaged.

This does not mean intellectual exercise. In fact, the brain does not function independently in this regard; the mind may very well be centered in the heart. The perception of the various internal organs in Traditional Chinese Medicine is based on a different concept than Western anatomy. Rather than seeing each organ as connected to its channel/meridian system like a radio to a car battery, we can look at the organs themselves as magnetic centers of energy that extend throughout the body through their function and channel system.

Tai Chi emphasizes the importance of the "third brain," the tan tien as an energetic and psychic center; but it is the heart that is "the heart." *Why* do we call the heart the heart? Were we to ask any group of educated or semi-educated people from the second grade onward in the United States the function of the heart, the overwhelming answer would be: "the heart pumps blood." Yet, all European languages consider the heart also the seat of emotion, the source of love. The heart is the center (from which we meditate), the heart of the matter, that which breaks too easily when confronted with what is perceived as overwhelming injustice, and is indeed where we love, and where we hate.

It is the Long Form that trains the heart.

CHAPTER 28.

YANG STYLE LONG FORM—

108 MOVEMENTS

FIRST SECTION

1. COMMENCEMENT--S

2. GRASP SPARROW'S TAIL LEFT-- SW

3. GRASP SPARROW'S TAIL RIGHT-- W

(ward-off, ROLLBACK, PRESS, PUSH)

4. SINGLE WHIP--E

5. PLAY THE HARP--S

6. WHITE CRANE SPREADS ITS WINGS—SE>E

7. BRUSH KNEE, TWIST STEP-E

8. PLAY GUITAR

9--11. BRUSH KNEE, LEFT, RIGHT, LEFT

12. PLAY GUITAR

13. BRUSH KNEE LEFT

14. STRIKE, PARRY, PUNCH

15. APPARENT CLOSE--S

16. CROSS HANDS

SECOND SECTION

17. CARRY TIGER OVER MOUN-TAIN—NW

18. PRESS & PUSH—NW

19. DIAGONAL SINGLE WHIP—SE>S>E

20. FIST UNDER ELBOW--E

21. REPULSE MONKEY, RIGHT

22. REPULSE MONKEY, LEFT

23. REPULSE MONKEY, RIGHT

24. DIAGONAL FLYING POSTURE--SW

25. PLAY THE HARP--S

26. WHITE CRANE COOLS ITS WINGS--E

27. BRUSH KNEE--E

28. NEEDLE AT SEA BOTTOM

29. FAN THROUGH BACK--S>W

30. TURN AND CHOP--W

31. STRIKE, PARRY, PUNCH

ACTIVATION

32. GRASP SPARROW'S TAIL, RIGHT

33. SINGLE WHIP--E

34. HANDS LIKE CLOUDS--S

35. HANDS LIKE CLOUDS

36. HANDS LIKE CLOUDS

37. SINGLE WHIP--E

38. HIGH PAT ON HORSE

39. SEPARATE RIGHT FOOT--E

40. SEPARATE LEFT FOOT

41. TURN, KICK WITH LEFT SOLE-- W

42. BRUSH KNEE, L

43. BRUSH KNEE, R

44. PUNCH DOWNWARD

45. FAN THROUGH BACK

46. TURN AND CHOP--N>E

47. STEP, PARRY, PUNCH--E

48. KICK WITH RIGHT FOOT

49. HIT TIGER, L--NW

50. HIT TIGER, R--SE

51. RIGHT HEEL KICK--E

52. PUNCH TO EARS--SE

53. LEFT HEEL KICK--E

54. TURN 360 degrees AND KICK RIGHT

55. STRIKE, PARRY, PUNCH

56. CROSS HANDS—S

THIRD SECTION

57. EMBRACE TIGER--NW

58. DIAGONAL SINGLE WHIP--SE

59. PART THE WILD HORSE'S MANE, R--W

61. WILD HORSE'S MANE, L

62. WILD HORSE'S MANE, R

63. GRASP BIRD'S TAIL, L--SW

64. GRASP BIRD'S TAIL, R--W

65. SINGLE WHIP--E

66. FAIR LADY AT THE SHUTTLES-- SW

67. FAIR LADY--SE

68. FAIR LADY--NE

69. FAIR LADY--NW

70. GRASP BIRD'S TAIL, L--SW

71. GRASP BIRD'S TAIL, R--W

72. SINGLE WHIP--E

73. WAVE HANDS LIKE CLOUDS--S

74. WAVE HANDS LIKE CLOUDS

75. WAVE HANDS LIKE CLOUDS

76. SINGLE WHIP—E

77. SNAKE CREEPS DOWN

78. GOLDEN COCK STANDS ON R. LEG

79. GOLDEN COCK STANDS ON L. LEG

80. REPULSE MONKEY

81. REPULSE MONKEY

82. REPULSE MONKEY

83. SLANTING FLYING--SW

84. PLAY THE HARP--S

85. WHITE STORK COOLS ITS WINGS--E

86. BRUSH KNEE

87. NEEDLE AT SEA BOTTOM

88. FAN THROUGH BACK>W

89. WHITE SNAKE STICKS OUT TONGUE

90. STRIKE, PARRY, PUNCH

91. GRASP BIRD'S TAIL, R

92. SINGLE WHIP--E

93. CLOUD HANDS--S

94. CLOUD HANDS

95. CLOUD HANDS

96. SINGLE WHIP--E

97. HIGH PAT ON HORSE

98. CROSS PALMS, TURN AND KICK>W

99. LOW BRUSH KNEE

100. LOW PUNCH

101. GRASP BIRD'S TAIL, R

102. SINGLE WHIP--E

103. SNAKE CREEPS DOWN

104. STEP UP, FORM SEVEN STARS

104. RETREAT TO RIDE TIGER

105. LOTUS KICK

106. SHOOT TIGER WITH BOW

107. STRIKE, PARRY, PUNCH

108. CROSS HANDS, CLOSE--S

Chapter 29.

Tai Chi Meditations:

"Commencement"

COMMENCEMENT is the first movement of the Yang Style Tai Chi Form. Though our discussion is of the essence rather than of the form, it is the form that gives Tai Chi its beauty and allure, its very being in the world. It is the form that is the vehicle for training the mind. The casual reader as well as the adept will then forgive a brief description of this movement for the express purpose of experiencing, in a limited way, the essence of Tai Chi Chuan.

EXERCISE #1. COMMENCEMENT

Commencement can hardly be called a movement, as the feet are kept in place, at shoulder width, with toes pointed directly forward (feet parallel to one another.) Knees slightly bent, and pointed with the toes. (For a more detailed description of the stance, see the "Horse Stance.")

As breath is guided into the lower abdomen—the Tan Tien area below the navel—the resultant sinking of weight, connected with the grounding of the body's energy through the feet, can be made to feel to raise the arms up in front of the body.

The arms are raised, directly in front of the body, with the joints soft, not locked, to a position parallel to the ground. In most forms, the palms face the ground. In Dr. Ho'o's Long Form, the palms face each other, activating the meridians in the arms and adding a variation in fighting applications. Dr. Ho'o describes the primalness of this stance as a mother reaching to child or child to mother. Sleepwalkers and ghosts in sheets have also been seen to use this position to advantage.

It is truly a simple, basic movement. Yet, we sometimes hear rumors of special Asian Tai Chi schools where this movement alone is practiced for the first six months of training. It is good to keep in mind the thought that true mastery of anything is mastery of the basics; those whom we consider to be masters are those who have found the depths of the simple things. "It's all right here," to paraphrase the Enlightened One. I think of John Coltrane—for all of his "sheets of sound," we always hear the basic chord progression, we always hear the blues. I think of Beethoven, cutting the needless details until the underlying musical form shined through like the light of heaven. I think of

Muhammad Ali, getting inside of so basic a thing as boxing to create art.

It all begins with the centering of the mind and body. And it all ends there. Though we have not yet taken a step, we have accomplished three very important steps on the road to increasing our levels of understanding of the integration of everything.

First, what happens in the movement? On the surface, the hands are raised. Dr. Ho'o's variation with the hands facing each other seems to activate the acupuncture/energy meridians, whereas the palms of the hands facing the ground is a more passive feeling, letting the earth herself fill and complete the movement.

Secondly, the body is double-weighted— what balances this? Where does the energy for raising the arms? Though this could be considered a movement that is not a movement and preliminary to the Form itself, double-weightedness is still something to be avoided.

Marshall Ho'o used to say, "Whatever comes up must come down." He talked a lot about reciprocity. Usually he meant, do one thing on one side of the body, and then do it on the other, for the health of the body and mind. However, there is a deeper meaning. What goes down when the arms come up?

When the body is relaxed and the arms seem to float upwards, there is the feeling they are being held by the back; we feel the activation in the lower-mid region. If we sink the energy into the tan tien and the weight through the feet into the ground, this seems to balance the double weighted aspect of this movement.

Thirdly, Commencement has another function: to balance the right and left sides of the body. We may be familiar with Ginshin-jitsu, or yogic breathing, which have a similar function. We can look at this two ways: either there are channels on the left and right sides of the body or the single channel has a left and right side which splits in the arms in and in the legs. In either case, our energy differentiates itself through left or right-handedness, through the natural distribution and often the health of organs in the body, through how we sit and work and many other factors. One side of the body has usually stronger energy; it is beneficial to use the stronger side to balance the weaker.

In Yogic breathing, we are dealing with and working with and through the upper body, through the breathing, which magnetizes the left and right currents. Or, according to the

Hindu texts, there are natural cycles where one side becomes activated, the other side passive. The method is to become independent of these cycles to promote health and longevity.

In Ginshin-jitusu we are holding the feet of another person. We are feeling the "pulse" of the energy and letting it travel through us, our right hand to their left foot; our left hand to their right; and sometimes crossing our arms.

When two people face each other—and this is true especially in a learning, healing or intimate situation, one on one—there is a subtle transference of energy because they are relating left to right, in opposite polarity.

With Commencement, we can feel the energy as if we are moving up a column of light; stabilizing it, root our feet, letting material energies fall to the center of the earth and our spiritual natures connect, in a very palpable way, through the Ba-Hui (crown of the head) to the infinity of the cosmos (Heaven). Many Tai Chi movements reflect the natural currents of the body—opposite in the upper and lower parts; but Commencement gives us an opportunity to address this flow directly.

Now, we are ready to move.

Chapter 30.

Tai Chi Meditations:

Grasp the Bird's Tail

The wind up and preparation for this movement—we call "say hello and hold the
ball"— is a deflection and strike to the
groin. We then take a step and raise the arm
into the "Peng" position. The arm up with
raised elbow—both in Grasp Bird's Tail
Left and also Ward Off (Grasp Bird's Tail
Right)—is typical of the Yang Style. It represents the wheel with the spine as the axle.
The action is one of deflection—direct force
upon the wheel either turns the wheel, bringing the force back upon the instigator; or,
one of compression. In the latter case, the
arm acts as not just part of a wheel, but part
of a sphere that absorbs force, then explo-
sively sends it back.

Traditionally, this movement is expressed
by the Hexagram Chen, the Creative—all
solid lines. The image is the dragon rising
in the fields; and there is indeed something
dragon-like about this posture, or the underlying feeling.

WARD OFF

In Ward Off we are first presented with the Great Secret; how to transmute energy. We are given the Lau-Kung point (Pericardium 4) on the right hand as the focal point for energy from the left hand. The left hand is the Yang hand in this instance, the weight being on the right foot. The right hand is empty, the rim of the wheel. This relates back to Chang San-Feng—his vision of the bird and the snake: the snake absorbs energy in a circular path instead of a direct retreat. Thus, it is able to absorb more energy than if it moved in a straight line.

The Yang aspect of Ward Off, like all the Tai Chi movements that shift from the rear foot to the front, is also performed in a circular, rather than straight-line fashion. This increases power by increasing distance traveled.

Playing with the math, $E = mc2$ means energy = mass times the speed of light squared.

This is undoubtedly a great deal of energy, because the speed of light (186,000 per second) is relatively fast. In Tai Chi, we are dealing with much slower speeds.

In space, very large distances are measured in terms of the light-year, which is the distance that light travels in a year (186,000 multiplied by 60x60x24x3651/4).   In Tai Chi, we are dealing with much smaller distances, but the difference in energy between bringing our weight forward in a straight line and in a circle is still significant.

Speed in general is defined as d/t, as in 50 miles per hour=50/1. That would mean one hundred miles in two hours is expressed as 100/2, which resolves to 50/1.

So, in our situation, we might express these relationships as

$E = md2$ (since time=1), that is

energy = weight times the square of the distance.

If we move the weight from one foot to the other, creating a radius of two feet, then that would make the circumference of the circle (pi times twice the diameter) 25 feet or so) and we have moved the hands at least on quarter of that distance. That would equal 43/4 feet, which means we have more than doubled our energy by circular movement.

If this method of computing energy is a little abstruse, consider the mechanics of the lever. The distance from the fulcrum is proportional to the weight that can be lifted with the same amount of energy. For example, with a 4-foot long lever, we can lift 200 pounds with 50 pounds of pressure. With an eight-foot lever, we can lift 400 pounds; which indicates again that distance traveled equals energy.

Transmuting Energy

What does it mean to transmute energy?

What is the difference between "chicken soup" of daily existence and the "living water" of the Holy spirit? There is no difference, really—just one of vibrational frequency. Why is the Hexagram representing "As Above, so Below" universal in philosophical systems? It is because the alchemical process, turning lead to gold, is ultimately suited to the human condition of being between Heaven and Earth, between the beasts of the field and angelic spheres.

Otherwise, all we are doing is moving our hands and feet around.

In learning Tai Chi Chuan, we are learning an art form; we must become aware not only of energy, but of vibrational quality of that energy. Not only are we increasing our energy potential by increasing distance externally, we are also becoming aware of increasing distance *internally* by raising frequency.

Turning lead to gold? Perhaps that is not the point. Perhaps we don't need to try to unlock all these "secrets" or to raise the human spirit to reach "higher" realms." We have found, from our study of the Law of Octaves, that vibrational frequency is a circle, or a spiral. The note A is 220, 440, 880, etc.; doubling at every octave. They are all difference A's, but still A.

Whatever and whoever we are, we are a vibrational frequency, and connected within a spiral of interlocking frequencies. As we know, a spiral is a very compact form; the DNA from a single human body, unwound from its spiral form, would reach to the moon and back 11 times.

Why does putting pieces of rock in concrete make it harder? It is surface area.

How many miles of shoreline in the world if we measure around every rock, every grain of sand?

In the previous volume, we discussed fractals; in the next volume, we will discuss Reflexology: how a small part of the body, such as the hand or foot or ear, contains an energetic replica of the entire body. It has been theorized that *every* part of the body, down to the smallest finger joint, comprises its own little universe, has a magnetic polarity, and reflects the entire body.

This gives new meaning to Dr. Ho'o's refrain: "When *one* part of the body moves, the *whole* body moves!"

In Tai chi, we are dealing with massive energy—the source of Yin and Yang, and we approach by the simplest and most concrete—something we learn (usually) by the time we are one year of age—transferring weight from one foot to the other in an upright position. After a while, we do not even think about how difficult those first few steps, keeping our balance, were; maybe we remember when we get to be 85 or 90. And we may also remember in Tai Chi class, where we learn to walk again, deconstructing and reconstructing the way we move, act and think.

Chapter 31. Some Tai Chi Principles

- Weight and energy sunk to the *tan t'ien* (center of gravity, psychic center and seed of movement two inches below the navel).

- Legs form inverted "U," not inverted "V."

- Knees bent--not locked, but never bent more than over the toe.

- Hands and feet do not move independently from each other, but together.

- (Rule of Three: always two hands and one foot in motion).

- "When one part of the body moves, the whole body moves".

- Head suspended, as from a string from heaven, spine like a string of pearls.

- Shoulders sunk (relaxed, not thrown back).

- The *chi* follows the mind, and the body follows the *chi.* (Keep eyes on the horizon, or slightly below, not down on ground).

- Elbows dropped (relaxed like they have weights attached to them).

- Wrist soft, fingers relaxed but extended, like Spanish roof tiles.
- Body and mind in state of relaxed attention *(sung)*

- Except for opening and closing, the Tai chi form is done with a clear division of *substantial* and *insubstantial*, usually a 70/30% division of weight. This not only strengthens the legs and activates the meridians (and immune system) but gives one more stability and maneuverability.

- There is a feeling of opening and pulling up in the back, and sinking in the chest.

- Breathing is coordinated with the rest of the body, yet natural. Do not focus on the breath, but generally, exhale on the more *Yang* movements.
- All movements should be smooth even and continuous. The energy ("jing") is not broken, but flows like water.

- Movements should be and appear effortless. There should be a feeling of aliveness (as opposed to "woodenness") in all parts of the body.

- If the left leg is empty, right arm is empty; if right leg is full, left arm is full.

- Movement in the legs generates energy, whereas movement of the arms calms.

- "Use four ounces to deflect 1000 pounds."

- This refers to awareness of energy, and the principle of deflection rather than blocking.

- The body should be erect and centered, leaning neither forward, backward, to the right or left. If pushed, the upper body "turns on an axle."

- "Tsou"--evasion or yielding. This is the Yin part of every movement. We are able to change instantly from attack to defense, and our thoughts should have the same flexibility. Yielding also implies *receptiveness.*

- "Chan"--sticking, adherence. This is practiced in push-hands, to always remain in contact with the opponent. It is a very effective fighting technique, since we are tuned in to his every movement and thought (research has demonstrated chemical changes in the skin when a person is thinking). "Sticking" also prevents an opponent from gathering momentum for a strike or push. It requires alertness and sensitivity.

- *Tai Chi*, the "Supreme Ultimate," is composed of Yin and Yang. When there is motion, the two separate. When there is stillness, the two recombine. In physics, we learn about *potential* and *kinetic energy*. (If I hold up a rock, for instance, that's potential; if I drop it, the energy becomes kinetic). Once energy is released, it becomes subject to different laws, and acts on matter differently. Though there is no absolute stillness within the form, there are relative stretches and contractions of the energy. It is an illusion that Yin and Yang are separate energies.

- One should be clear about the distribution of weight and energy in the body. It is instructive to analyze how Yin and

Yang interact and change with each movement of the Form; one should be able to change instantly.

- Movements should be smooth, with no speeding up or slowing down. Each movement should be distinct, with a definite beginning and ending, yet there should be no break in the energy (the essence of unwinding a silk thread from a cocoon).

- Movements should be and appear effortless. There should be a feeling of aliveness (as opposed to "woodenness") in all parts of the body.

- Mind is neither on the breath nor the chi, but on the spirit (*shen*). *Chi* is stored (in the bones) and let go. It is stored like the bending of a bow (curved) and released like shooting an arrow (straight).

- Movement in the feet and legs generates energy, whereas movement of the hands and arms is calming.

- Keep the mind quiet and smooth: still, when the body is in motion and active, when the body is still. This is the basis of body/mind awareness. It is similar to the mechanism of a clutch in a standard transmission: concentration is *shifted* when motion is begun--the mind unifies with the energy and does not interfere with the flow of movement.

- Except for opening and closing, the Tai chi form is done with a clear division of *substantial* and *insubstantial*, usually a 70/30% division of weight. This not only strengthens the legs and activates the meridians (and immune system) but gives one more stability and maneuver-ability.

- The body should be erect and centered, leaning neither forward, backward, to the right or left.

Chapter 32. The Five Downs

1. THE SHOULDERS: At no time should the shoulders be raised in Tai Chi. "Commencement" is a good movement in which to practice raising the arms and keeping shoulders relaxed. Tension in the shoulders blocks energy from the spine through the arms. Note how raising the shoulders changes not only energy, but psychic state and the center of gravity.

2. THE ELBOWS: The elbows should feel as if hung with heavy weights, then they will be relaxed even in those movements when they do come up, such as "White Stork Cools its Wings." Do each movement in the form while paying attention to the elbows. Tension in the elbows changes the dynamics, the

form and the energy flow from the shoulders.

3. THE HEELS: Having the heel come up when weight is shifted from that foot is an indication of too high a center of gravity, and not being grounded. The heel should be down unless all weight is coming off the foot in preparation for a step.

4. THE BUTTOCKS: The lower back must be in a straight line, the buttocks tucked under rather than pushed out or cocked to the side. The hips should be parallel to the ground. This is important for proper posture and movement.

5. THE WEIGHT AND ATTENTION: At the same time as the head is suspended, the weight of the body sinks straight into the ground. Rather than creating a feeling of heaviness, it is a feeling of relaxation, alertness and power coming from the earth. The attention should also be relaxed, though alert, and sunk to the Tan Tien, two or three inches below the

navel. This is not only the center of gravity and of movement, but is the psychic center of the human organism. The *tan tien,* rather than the brain, is capable of awareness of the present moment.

Chapter 33.

YANG'S TEN IMPORTANT POINTS:

Discussion of principles of Yang, Chen-Fu

1. The head should be upright so the shen can reach the headtop

EXERCISE: Standing in Horse Stance (knees bent slightly, legs forming inverted U shape); draw (an imaginary) line from the back of the ears to the center of the head—the midpoint of that line is the Ba-hui. Imagine being pulled up from this point. The eyes stay just below the line of the horizon. Sink the energy and all material force through the feet into the ground, the non-material energy rises and we are 'suspended from heaven.'

Perhaps this is what is meant by humankind being 'between heaven and earth.' In our Western tradition, we partake of the nature of both "the angels of heaven and the beasts of the field." That is who we are. The word *material* comes from the Latin root mater (mother). This is the feminine, grounding force. The opposing, complementary male force holds us up. The Western tradition speaks of a "silver cord connecting us to Heaven."

Where is Heaven?

It is easy for Westerners to be confused by the term *heaven*. We may think of it as a place to go after the transition of death. However, the concept also occurs in Hebrew cosmology—man being between the angels of heaven and the beasts of the field. In reality, we are not just connected to the earth; we are a part of her, just as "the beasts of the field." We are actually a part of heaven also. There is part of us that does not exist on the plane of the earth. We are not only "connected" to heaven through the "silver cord" from the Ba-Hui—we are part of heaven. This concept of heaven is not to be confused with what the birds fly around in or where we may or may not go when we die. This heaven is, if not particularly tangible, an operational part of our existence.

The practice of Tai Chi Chuan helps us to tune in to these two forces, Yin and Yang. These forces are with us with every movement, with every breath; they have existed literally since the birth of this universe.

The original meaning of the word Tai Chi was "ridgepole." The ridgepole of a house holds the two sides of the roof together. This very concrete application of the principle of connecting opposites became the abstract notion of anything that connects two opposites.

In order for us to move at all, we are involved with this division of Yang and Yin. In terms of movement, we call this "full and empty," or "weighted and unweighted."

We may interpret " ridgepole" as the spine, but it is even more the sense that Yin and Yang are in continuous change and fluctuation from one side to the other; there is something that does not change, that stays in the center, in control.

Tai Chi has a natural rootedness, but is not stiff or wooden. It is the continuous flow of Yin and Yang that gives life to the movements. One thinks of the feeling and spirit of gymnasts and Wu Shu acrobats; there is a "sparkle" to their movements, elasticity. This comes from being in peak physical condition after years of work. It would not hurt anyone to imitate their demeanor, their joy and seriousness. Confidence comes from practice and understanding, as opposed to what one might think of as "natural," which is merely conditioned.

For instance, the natural reaction when confronted with force is to use force back, or to tense up. This conditioned response is deep, but not irreversible. Using force, referred to as *li* in the Classics, produces tension that stops the flow of energy.

Usually, both hands are kept moving slightly throughout the form. All parts of the body are relaxed, "sung." Additionally, we must remember the principle that all movement is connected; for example, the head or arms will not move independently of the rest of the body. "When one part of the body moves, the whole body moves."

2. Sink the chest and pluck up the back.

EXERCISE: Standing two feet from a wall, lean until your hands, about heart level, are resting on the wall with the weight of your body. Pull back up from this position without using the strength of your arms. Pull from the Ming-mung, mid-back, opposite the Tan-tien. This will naturally straighten the curve of the back, pulling the spine outward and depressing the chest.

The rootedness of the entire body is dependent upon not sticking out the chest. At the same time, we should not be hunched over or appearing weak. Though a weak stance is a useful ploy in combat to make others underestimate our skill, the point of sinking the chest is not to look like a bedraggled chicken. The spine, in a natural, relaxed position, is slightly curved; by straightening it, we are storing energy, much like pulling back on the string of a bow.

One can think of Fa-ching not as a special force, but a special focusing of energy. Everyone has had the rare experience of doing something perfectly. Perhaps this was by accident—almost always "without thinking," and invariably "without trying." In our daily existence, we may notice things such as a perfectly hit billiard ball, a wadded paper thrown in the trash; perhaps there are perfect things that go unnoticed.

Though this kind of perfection in very small things is not as uncommon as one might think, it is less common to see a whole poem that is perfected, or a novel or a symphony. For a whole life to be perfected is a miracle. Those people are extremely rare. Yet perfection is a matter of perspective—in a sense, we are all perfect. How can we not be? An imperfection in a single leaf in a tree is imperceptible to an observer across the street; even a broken limb on a single tree is not noticed by an observer of the entire forest from a distant hillside. The moreness or lessness of perfection is minuscule, compared to the infinite perfection of the Infinite, of which we are all a part.

Depressing the chest and plucking up the back also relates to the circulation of internal energy and breathing techniques. The concept of the macrocosmic orbit was popularized in the books of Mantak Chia, but previously mentioned by Professor Wen Shan Huang in his (still out of print) book The Fundamentals of Tai Chi Chuan, and discussed by Carl Jung in The Secret of the Golden Flower. In China, people have been practicing it for hundreds of years. It is the author's belief that the culmination of this type of practice is responsible for the many tales from China and India of miraculous feats.

The energy circulates naturally up the spine to the head. East Indian practice calls this the Kundalini energy. The image is of a snake uncoiling. When practicing, it may be more effective to "tune in" to this energy, rather than "visualize." This energy exists whether we are visualizing it or not. The point may not be to increase or control the energy as much as to focus the attention and intent by concentrating the mind on something so subtle.

Practice of internal energy may result in unusual sensations or states of consciousness. However, Tai Chi is a "middle way" practice. The goal is ordinary consciousness with extraordinary clarity, or to accomplish ordinary tasks with exceptional skill. The rising of the energy to the head may be pleasant, or powerful—the headdresses, or eagle feathers of Native people express the beauty of this energy. The Tai Chi way is to remain rooted, focused and connected, no matter what occurs or seems to occur.

Once the energy travels up the spine to the head, in the acupuncture meridian we call the Governing Vessel, it travels down the face, into the mouth over the head, around the nose and into the mouth. There, the tongue connects, by a light pressure just behind the upper front teeth, to the Conception Vessel, which runs down the front of the body to the perineum. There, it again connects again to the Governing Vessel. This circle or circuit is known as the Microcosmic Orbit.

One can use "reverse breathing" or "Taoist breathing" to aid in this circulation by pushing the energy up the back. This is accomplished in the following manner: bring the air deep into the lungs, filling the lower abdomen; however, instead of extending or protruding the abdomen, depress those muscles as if you were forcing the air up the back. Exhaling, tighten and extend the lower belly, pushing the energy downward.

This technique is also called "pre-natal breathing," as it resembles how a fetus in a womb sucks air through the umbilicus. This type of breathing may seem unnatural; however, when punching, pushing, or otherwise involved in extreme exertion, we may automatically tighten and push out the abdominal muscles while exhaling.

3. Sung (relax) the waist.

We now translate "waist" as the Kwa, that area between the legs and the groin. It is likely that the original translation of Kwa as waist was probably made by a British translator; the British concept of waist can be the entire upper body—as in waistcoat. The word Kwa and concept is relatively new in the West.

There is another Tai chi saying: the power, or energy, "comes from the legs, is controlled by the waist (kwa) and is expressed by the hands." Thus, the Kwa is the controller, or commander. In our culture or mindset, we tend to think of the brain as the controller. For us to give up control to a part of our bodies that is not the brain may be outside of our comfort zone. However, it may be something we do unconsciously rather frequently.

The Kwa transfers the energy from the lower to the upper body. We note that doing certain movements may be more difficult on one side that the other. In throwing a ball, for instance, what gives the movement its power and fluidity is the connection of the lower and upper body. Some talented athletes seem to be born with this ability. Others of us have to work on it. Tai Chi is excellent for anyone undertaking any athletic or other activity that requires muscular co-ordination. By training slowly, we can change habits of movement that solidified even at the age of five or six years of age. Not only can great athletic ability be developed, if that is one's goal, but there is room for improvement in both the least and the most talented.

By connecting the lower and upper body, the Kwa is important in achieving maximum effect of upper body movements. In our practice of the form, we learn to move the body as a whole, and not to use the arms and upper body by itself. We focus on using mind instead of strength, using the weight instead of muscular strength, and utilizing the lower body to empower the upper. The martial artist Bruce Lee developed a powerful "one-inch punch," which was able to stun or knock out opponents. Undoubtedly, part of its efficacy was in folding and un-folding of the Kwa, as the distance of the punch is then increased exponentially. It has been purported that his favorite exercise was Advance and Retreat.

The Kwa area contains over 50 lymph nodes, the largest collection in the body. The Chinese, refer to the legs as "the second heart," because of their ability to pump the lymph. The lymph is a clear, colorless liquid that has the job of detoxifying the tissues of the body. Actually, the lymphatic system runs throughout the body, and has four important functions:

1. By connecting the tissues with the circulatory system, it removes excess fluids.

1. absorbs fatty acids and subsequent transport of fat to the circulatory system
2. produces immune cells, such as lymphocytes, monocytes, and antibody-producing cells.
3. contains white blood cells, preventing viral or bacterial infections

The lymph, as well as moving by low pressure peristalsis, is pumped by skeletal muscles, and contains one-way valves, and various points in the body that connect to the circulatory system. Thus, the use of the Kwa in Tai Chi Chuan has the added benefit of activating these important functions. We have noted elsewhere that Tai Chi is a significant activator of the immune system, as well as a powerful component of weight-loss programs.

EXERCISE: GRINDING CORN (as described in Chapter 25)

With legs double shoulder width apart, squat down, knees over toes, back straight, arms in front (palms down) in circular motion on the lateral plane. Shift weight from left to right, folding Kwa.

Reverse the circles.

4 Differentiate insubstantial and substantial.

 This is the Tai Chi symbol,

otherwise known as the Yin/Yang symbol. We know that it symbolizes the polar, complementary opposites of which the universe, in all manifestations, partakes. Stepping back for a moment from Chinese philosophy, examining Hindu philosophy can shed further light upon this concept.

One of India's most ancient and revered texts is The Bhagavad-Gita. Chapter Fourteen speaks of the three gunas: sattva, rajas and tamas. They stand respectively for wisdom, action and ignorance. Quoting from the Gita:

The three gunas, born of Nature—

Sattva, rajas and tamas—

bind to the mortal body

the deathless embodied Self.

Of these three, sattva, untainted,

luminous, free from sorrow,

binds by means of attachment

to knowledge and joy, Arjuna.

Rajas is marked by passion,

born of craving and attachment;

it binds the embodied Self

to never-ending activity.

Tamas, ignorance-born,

deludes all embodied beings;

it binds them, Arjuna, by means of

dullness, indolence and sleep.

And from Chapter Three:

No one, not even for an instant,

can exist without acting; all beings

are compelled, however unwilling,

by the three strands of Nature called gunas

If we were to see wisdom and ignorance as opposites, action is what is created by their interaction.

Back to Chinese thought, the empty circle symbolizes Wei Chi, the Unmanifest, Tai Chi being the Manifest, the division into Yin and Yang, which occurs with the least movement or thought. In the language of quantum physics, the quantum field collapses when energy (in the form of thought or directionality) is applied to the field. The analogue becomes the digital, the infinite the finite.

In the Tai Chi Chuan form, this is expressed in the first movement, Commencement; here, stillness becomes movement in the vertical and sagittal planes. Then, as the body turns, in all three dimensions.

The division of Yin and Yang is made clear by the shift of weight. Never in the form, except for the beginning and end of each section of the Long Form, and possibly as a transitory state, is weight equal in both feet. Double-weightedness is to be avoided.

We have noted elsewhere that weightedness is opposite in the upper and lower body. If the right leg is weighted, or energized, the left hand is energized; if the right leg is empty, then the right hand is full, the left hand empty. This concept promotes an extra level of balance in the body, and promotes the flow of energy throughout the body. Awareness of substantiality and insubstantiality also help us to move more quickly and smoothly.

EXERCISES:

Advance and Retreat adding the hands. This is called Reeling Silk. Unwinding of the silk cocoons is so delicate a process that it used to be done only by children. The silk must be unwound in a straight line or the fragile threads may break. First, with weight on the right foot, hold the ball over the right knee. Based on our knowledge of martial arts, we know this is a hit to the groin; therefore, the left hand is on the bottom, and weighted as we begin Retreat to the left. As we shift to the left foot, the right hand becomes heavy and falls, and we are now on the left foot, holding the ball with the left hand on top of the ball. The entire movement can also be reversed (see Warm-Up Exercises: Advance)

There is, in Tai Chi Chuan, an important concept known as "grinding the heel." We know that weight is to be taken off the moving foot, to promote ease and to take strain off the knee. We know to be careful practicing on carpets and on the bare earth. There may be some weight left in the foot, but this could hardly be called "grinding the heel." It is the author's opinion at that grinding the heel refers to the foot with the weight. You feel it in the Kwa, for instance the left kwa, which is full; it opens as you turn right and closes as you turn left. It is that weighted left heel that grinds as you move. This is important, as otherwise you might think that that side of the body, since it is not moving, is actually static. It is not. The energy is moving there as much as the side that is turning. Let us not forget the hands—the right hand is also "grinding," or performing some kind of energetic action appropriate to its dimensional energetic activity. In addition, consider the opposite of "grinding"— possibly "floating," or, "unwinding."

5. Sink the shoulders and elbows.

Raising the elbows tenses the shoulders. Tensing the shoulders means that the energy will not flow. If the energy does not flow, we are cut off from our source of power, *unbroken* force   connected with the infinite. This is true power, unbeatable and unstoppable. Whether the energy is for fighting or healing, or fighting/healing, we are careful that the force is coming through us rather than from us; the alternative is dissipation of our intrinsic energy.

If the mind is in confusion, the brain is overactive, and the energy remains too high in the body. Puffing out the chest, raising the nose and chin too high, besides being parodies of excessive pride, indicate weakness. It can also be dangerous: one's health can be adversely affected by wrong be adversely affected by wrong posture; additionally, having energy centered in places other than the Tan Tien can result in accidental injuries.

Feeling the infinite is usually a result of being centered. The natural, rather than the altered state of consciousness is connection with the infinite. We may not recognize it as such because our minds are tied with so many conscious and unconscious and semi-conscious strings to our environment—"the tree of life whose roots are in heaven and whose branches reach down and engulf us," to paraphrase the Bhagavad Gita.

EXERCISE: YOGIC BREATHING. Actualize the concept of "offering the inhalation to the exhalation"; and then the "exhalation to the inhalation."

6. Use mind and not force.

*T*he book <u>Power vs. Force</u> is a unique work that uses muscle testing, which is related to radiosthenics, or dowsing, to objectively rate the energy level of any particular idea, person, place or thing. The author makes a distinction between force (li) and power (i), which of course rates higher. The difference is that (i) is a spiritual power connected with the universe; li, on the other hand, is a distortion, an ego-driven assertion of finite power that can be easily overcome. In a commentary on Yang Chen-Fu's work by Chen Wei Ming, we have an important clue to the production of internal power. We are told not to fill up the acupuncture channels with the lower form of energy, to keep them clear and empty; we are advised not to let our energy float, and, when we do use strength, not to let it show.

However, *i* is not a purely mental force or power, just as *li* is not purely mental. It is not enough to involve the brain, just as it is ineffective to merely visualize the result with no physical involvement. With *i*, we go beyond the mental and physical into the realm where they merge.

That is where our practice comes in. The emptying/clearing of channel is part of our continuous practice. We are given the gift of daily challenges, obstacles to overcome. If we are given no obstacles, then that situation is, indeed, a challenge. For most of us, there are daily obstacles, and there is usually a right way and a wrong way to deal with them. Common sense will give us the answer, if our awareness is "turned on."

The problem for many of us is *overload*. Just as when the body becomes overloaded, our mind can become toxic and we can fall into unwanted, unskillful ways of interacting with the world, or even with our own minds.

Awareness of our own state of mind is one of the keys, and one of the very exciting benefits of Tai Chi practice.

EXERCISE: Do Tai Chi one entire day, just living your life as normal with the difference that you are using Tai Chi to perform every movement, solve every challenge.

7. Upper and lower mutually follow.

We have discussed the use of the waist (kwa) as connection between the lower and upper body; also, the first chapter of this volume relates the relaxing of the middle portion of the body to the I-Ching. We have discussed the microcosmic orbit—the flow of energy up the spine, over the head, then down of the body to the perineum and back around. The Macrocosmic Orbit is similar, but it comes all the way from the feet, or from the ground through the feet.

EXERCISE:

On the inhalation, bring the energy from K-1, THE BUBBLING SPRING, up the inside of the legs to the groin area where the two channels cross and go up the back, then down the yang side (outside) of the arms at the same time as over the head, down the face and into the mouth.

On the exhalation, the energy travels from the upper palate behind the front teeth through the tongue down the front of the body, at the same time from the fingers across the yin side of the arms (inside), crossing again at the groin area and going down the outside of the legs and feet and back into the ground.

In this context, *the body is the teacher.* Wherever we are, that is where we are. Just being in our bodies….think of playing music. You are a soloist in a band. You wait your turn, listening intently to the music— swimming in it, but keeping your place automatically. Suddenly, it is your turn. You're ready, you know the song, you understand the rhythm, the groove and the harmonic structure of your environment. It is impossible to play a wrong note; you even try to play a wrong note and you laugh hat how easily you fall back on track. You play one note at a time, even if thinking and feeling in shapes; but the note you're on is the note you're *on.* You are tied physically to that note, and when you've moved on, you are somewhere else.

8. Inside and outside coordinate.

The process of completion is carried out with the mind and body intact—in this life-time, as it were. We are still doing the form but it is now on a different level. Tai Chi is an art. This is the subject of Volume Three of this series: Completion.

Art is the process of balancing inside and outside. The nature of the human mind is such that we see everything that occurs on the outside on an "inner screen." Artistic expression is one way we can flip the screen around, or turn ourselves inside-out.

As this expressiveness becomes merged with the self, as it becomes a commitment and a way of life, then an *inner life* develops. It is almost as if another self is created. Words seem inadequate to describe this process.

EXERCISE: Doing any familiar part of the form, be aware of every part of the body— down to the separate joints of the fingers and toes— as having its own polarity, its own reflexiveness to the body as a whole and the movement as a whole.

9. It is mutually joined and unbroken.

It is perhaps ironic that the very elements within our lives we wish to control or eliminate we can eventually see as great gifts. Often, this is the work of a lifetime; it is what is really happening as the rest of our lives is taking place. Esoteric texts describe the "Great Work"—raising the frequency of energy on this planet and in this universe. There is no one of us that is not part of that effort; there are no lost moments or wasted time.

A leaf falls from a tree. Were we waiting for it, we could not predict the moment. We also cannot put it back once it has fallen. Yet, within this single dimensional, linear time-frame, we must create meaning—but only for *ourselves*. It is not necessary to be able to explain it to others. They'll get it, if you believe it, or if you're real about it.

The river flows downstream. Yet, there has to be water upstream for the flow to exist or continue. In the great mind of the universe, the energy is carried both ways.

EXERCISE: As we previously offered inhalations to exhalations, as per Yogic breathing, we will now offer the Yang part of a movement to the Yin part. If we are careful to prepare the movement by placement of the foot in advance of shifting of the weight, the result should be unparalleled smoothness of movement.

10. Seek stillness in movement.

Most people learn to relax in a Push Hands context within a few minutes. For the training to carry over into daily life may require much more than one or two classes. It is more difficult to learn this on ones own. It is invaluable experience to have these classes. However, once one realizes the principles and has developed some self control, it is possible to "practice' within the conflictual confines of daily life.

Push Hands principles can be used in at least three ways. We must consistently seek to discover and re-discover these principles in actual Push Hands practice. This is the process of training the mind to train the body. The goal of this may not be to train the body at all, but to train the mind. It is an indirect method; direct methods of training the mind are often problematic and by definition, always circular.

Once the mind has been trained, even slightly, then one behaves differently in the world. Interactions on all levels loose their emotional charge and become vehicles for more training and practice.

The third area that push hands practice is invaluable is within the mind itself. Applying Push Hands principles of yielding and not meeting force with force is useful in "quieting the mind;" indeed, it is the only method possible.

EXERCISE:

Sink the chi to the tan tien. To accomplish this, use the mind and use the breath…just the mind and the breath.

Jeffrey Fisher

Known nationally and internationally as an award-winning composer, master musician, painter and lecturer, Jeffrey Fisher has been a writer since the age of nine, and started cooking at the age of five. He attended Pomona College as a Theatre/Eastern Philosophy student, and studied music and composition at SUNY at Buffalo and the Grove School, Studio City. Fisher's first exposure to Tai Chi Chuan was at NYU School of the Arts and later studied under Master Y.C. Chiang in Berkeley and Dr. Marshal Ho'o in California, as well as with many of Dr. Ho's students.

Fisher now lives on and maintains an off-the-grid retreat in the San Jacinto Mountains, practices Reflexology and Auricular Medicine, teaches Tai Chi Chuan, writes and plays the flute and bass violin. His four albums: Triumph of the Spirit, Fairy Tales – from the Ballet Hans Christian Andersen, Ocean of Consciousness, and Satyagraha – Songs of the Earth are all available on order from many of the large and small retailers; as are the following volumes of White Cloud Journey: The Tao of Just About Everything and Completion. www.HealingMusicoftheSouthwest.com, www.twobirdsflying.com.

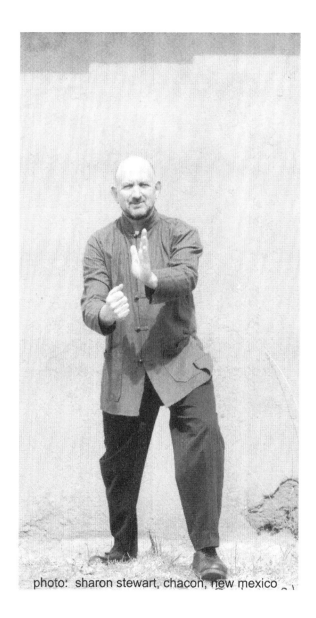

photo: sharon stewart, chacon, new mexico

8439785R0

Made in the USA
Charleston, SC
09 June 2011